Sofat and Sobrat's Island Discovery

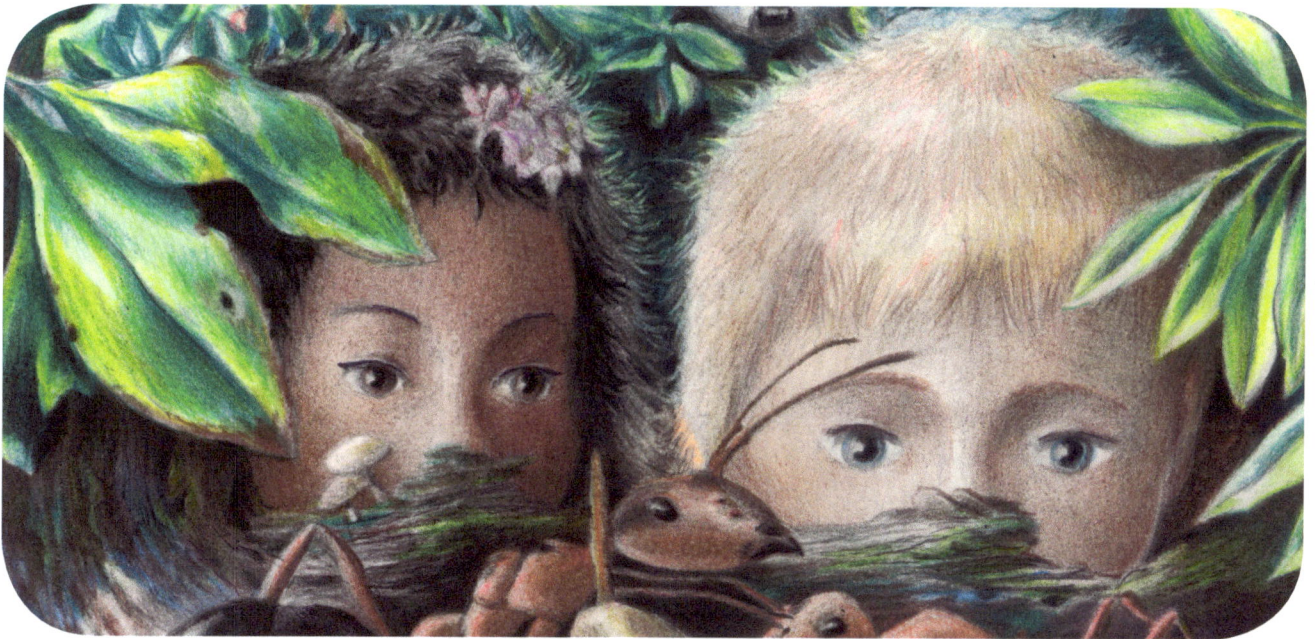

WRITTEN AND ILLUSTRATED BY

ALAN M HINES

Toddlers to Dodderers Publishing

Dedicated to

A More Fit and Thoughtful World

Toddlers to Dodderers Publishing

Picture-Perfect Tales for All Ages

Visit Us Online

www.toddlerstododdererspublishing.com

Email: t2dpublishing@att.net

Also by Alan Hines

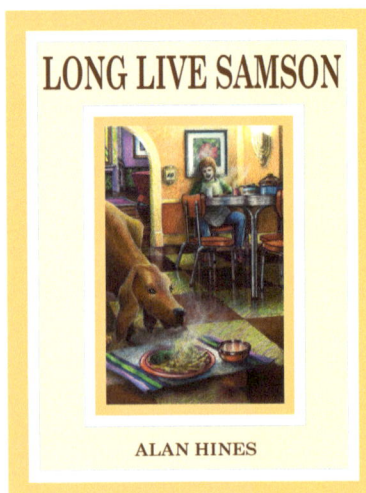

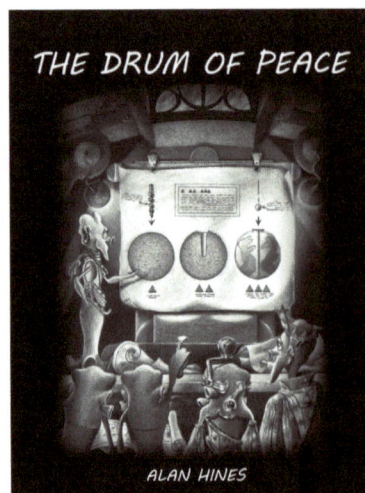

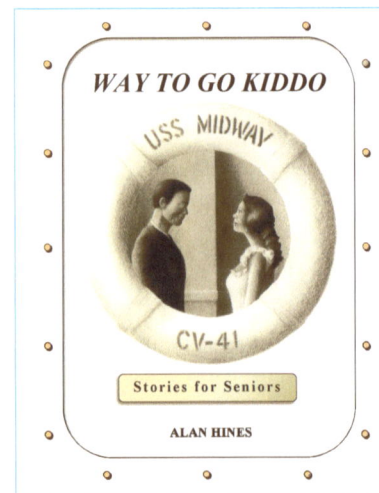

LONG LIVE SAMSON

ALAN HINES

THE DRUM OF PEACE

ALAN HINES

WAY TO GO KIDDO

USS MIDWAY

CV-41

Stories for Seniors

ALAN HINES

Sofat and Sobrat's Island Discovery

Ready for an adventure?

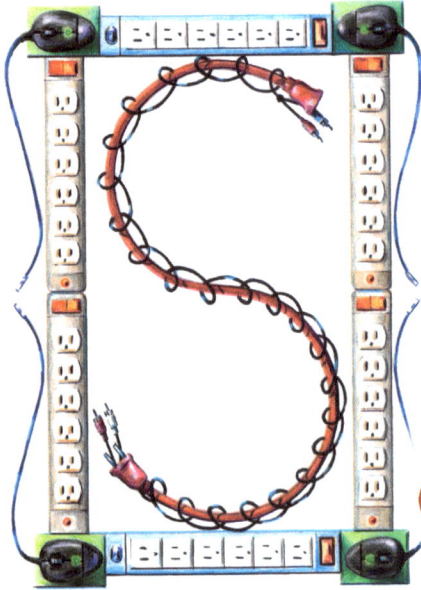

Sofat and **Sobrat** had so much it seemed; such as games, goodies and houses that gleamed. Whatever they asked for, their parents would buy. Their toys and computers could pile to the sky.

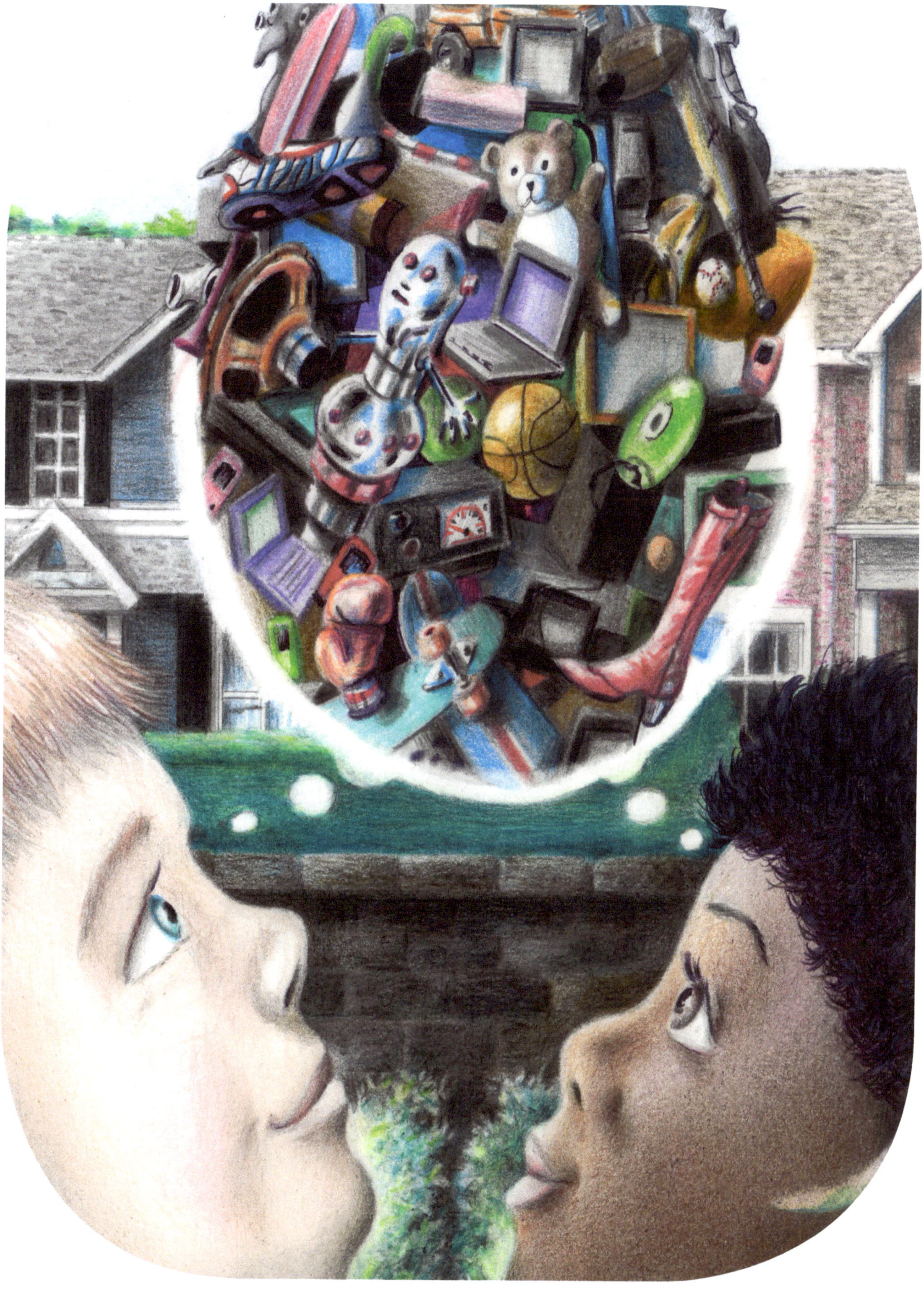

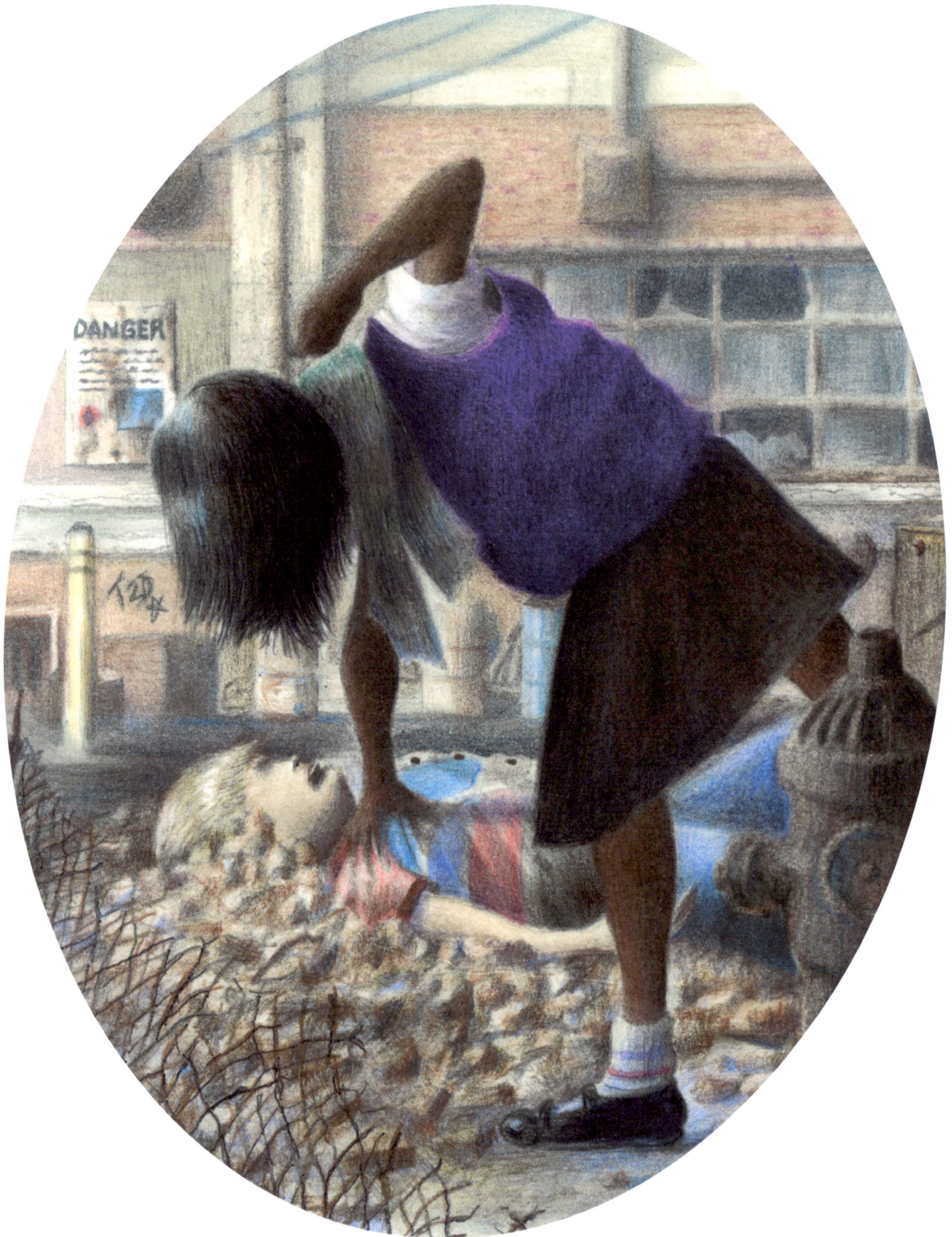

Sobrat did bully and was a loose nut.

Sofat was lazy and sat on his butt.

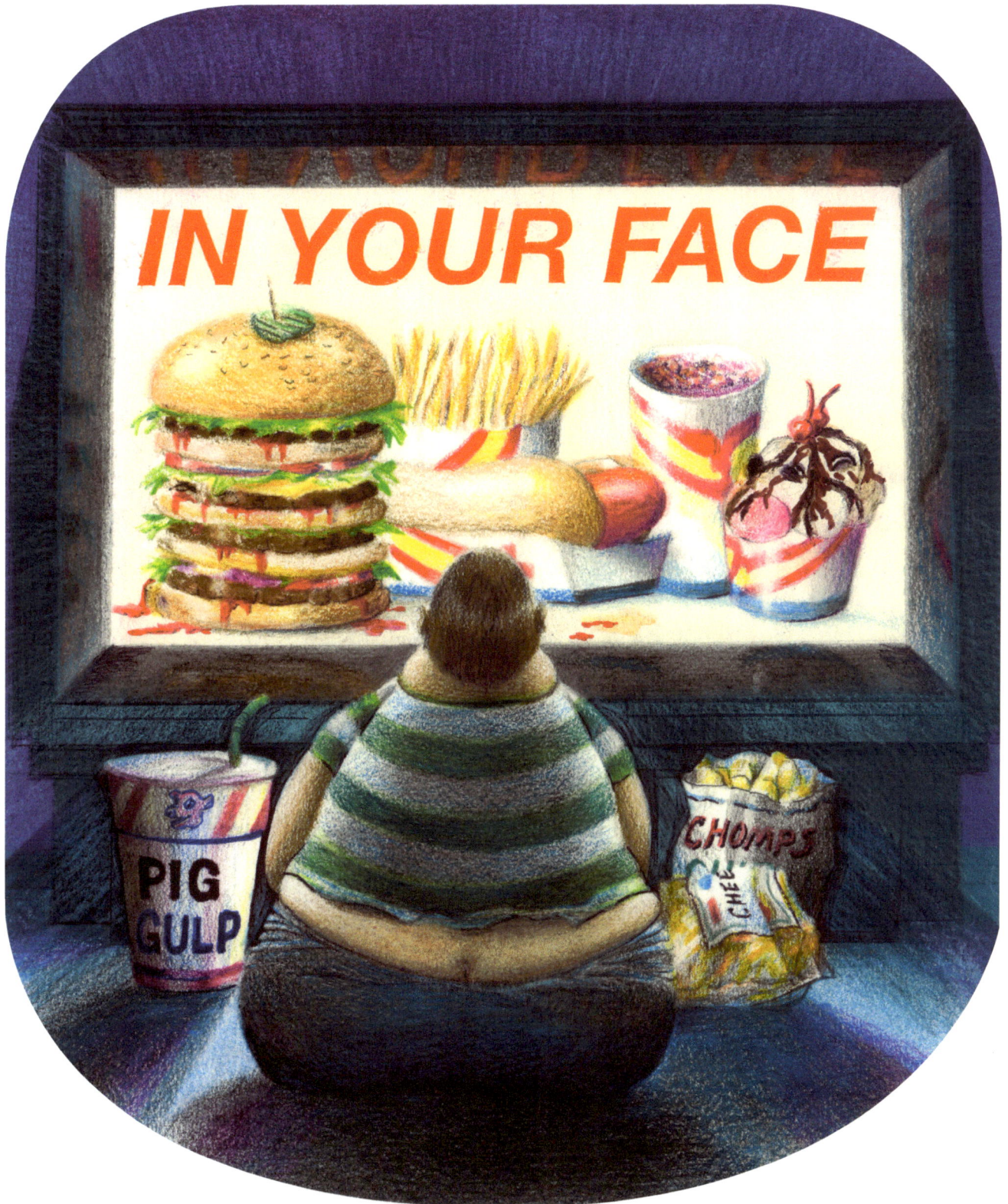

Spoiled as could be, they thought they were cool;
but both were just like their classmates at school.

They were slaves to devices and gadgets with frills.
These toys made them sharp, but dulled people skills.

Their peers played with phones, pads, and cameras with zoom, while completely ignoring their friends in the room.

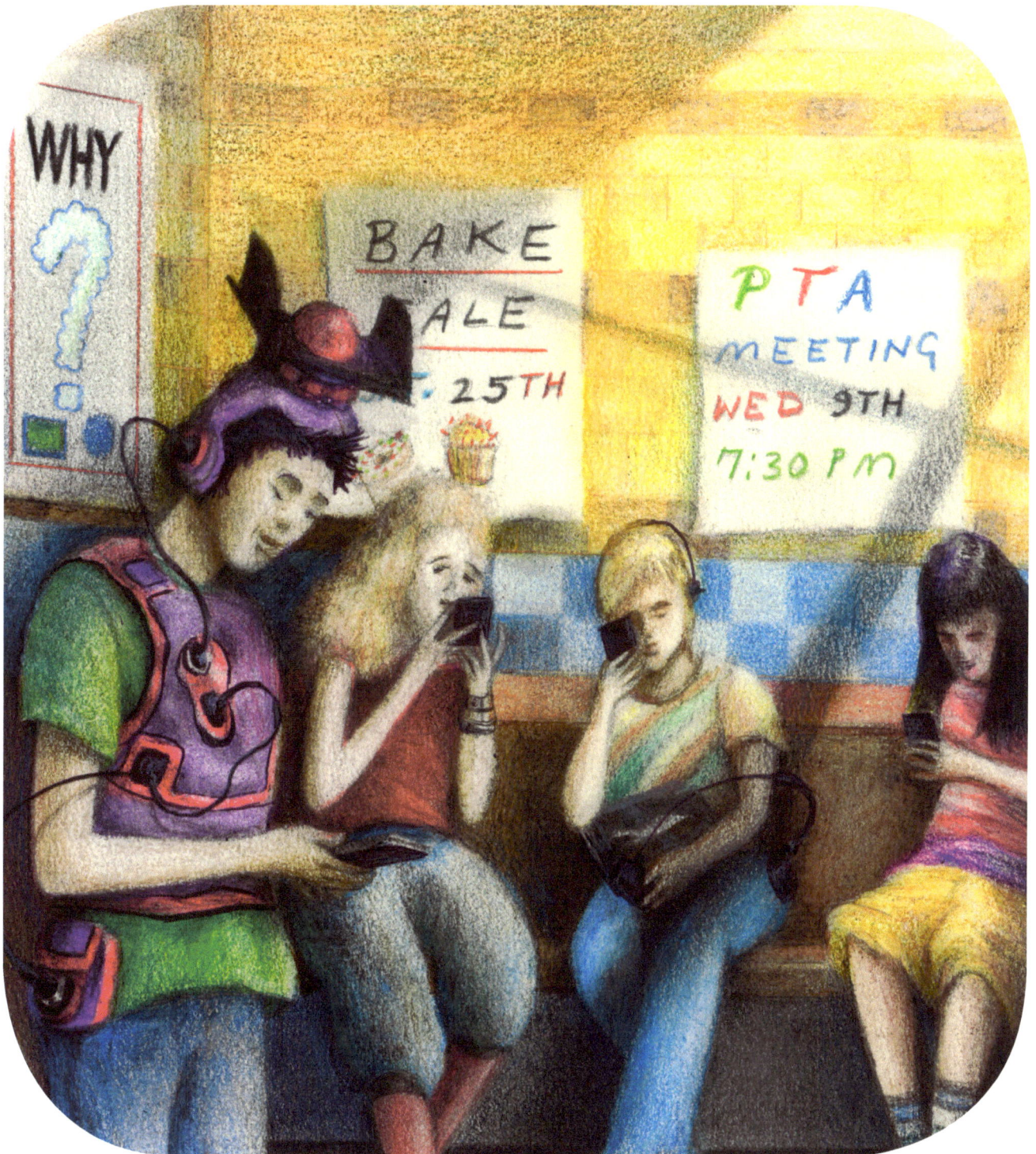

When boredom set-in the two built a raft. It held lots of snack bags and was a fine craft.

The vessel was launched in a beautiful lake.
Sofat had grabbed loads of snack food to take.

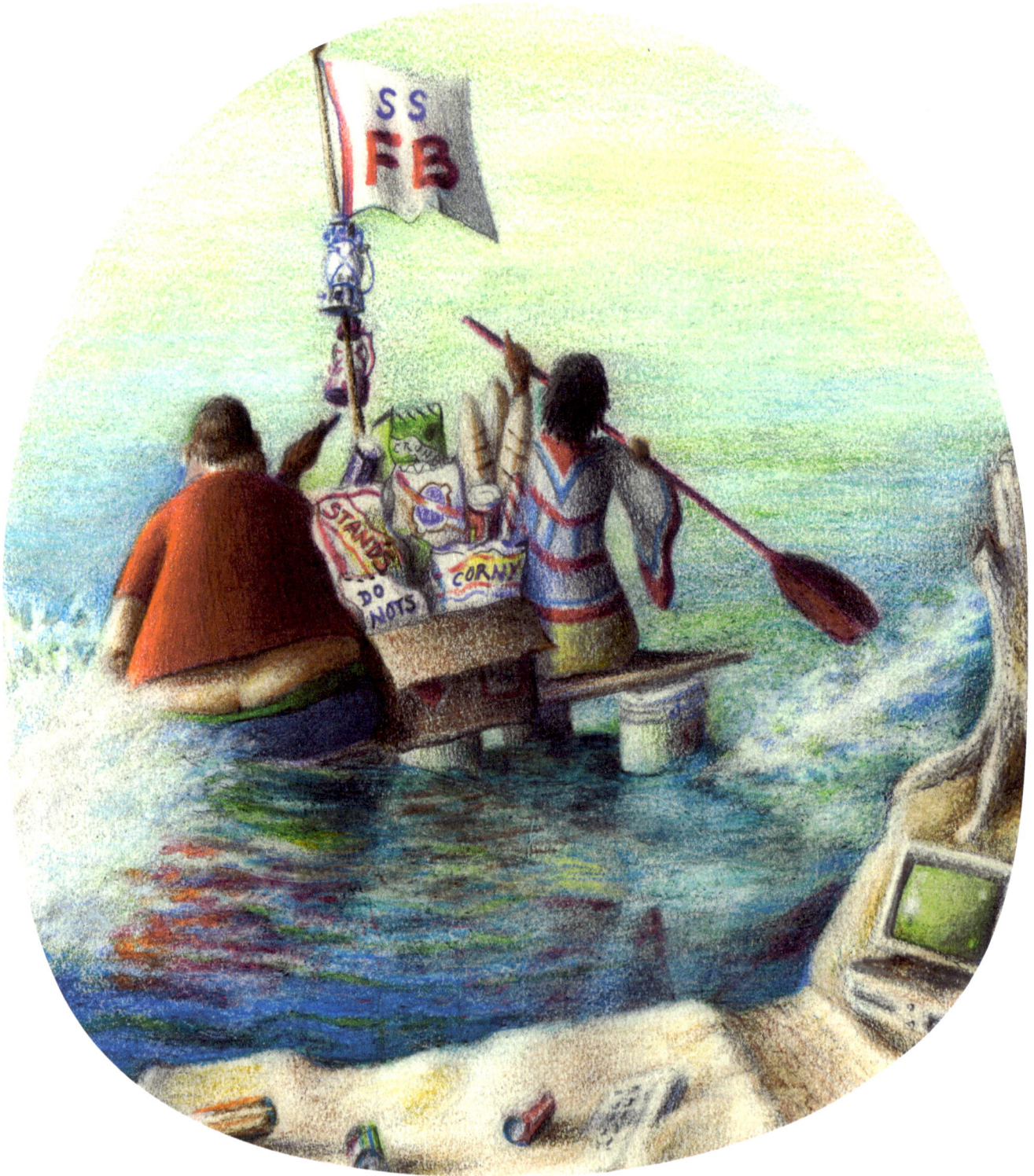

Sobrat brought games and stuff she might use.
If things became drab, these things would amuse.

She also had lanterns and other supplies,
in case of bad weather or some big surprise.

They paddled with might and raced far from shore.
Sofat was soft, so his muscles grew sore.

After a time no land could be seen.
The water was deep and a pretty blue-green.

Sobrat was hungry and snatched up a snack.
Sofat got angry and gave her a whack. "That's my
food," he scoffed as he took back his candy.
"Just keep your paws off and things will stay dandy."

"That's fine," she exclaimed, "but I won't share my stuff."
She then turned away in a whimsical huff.

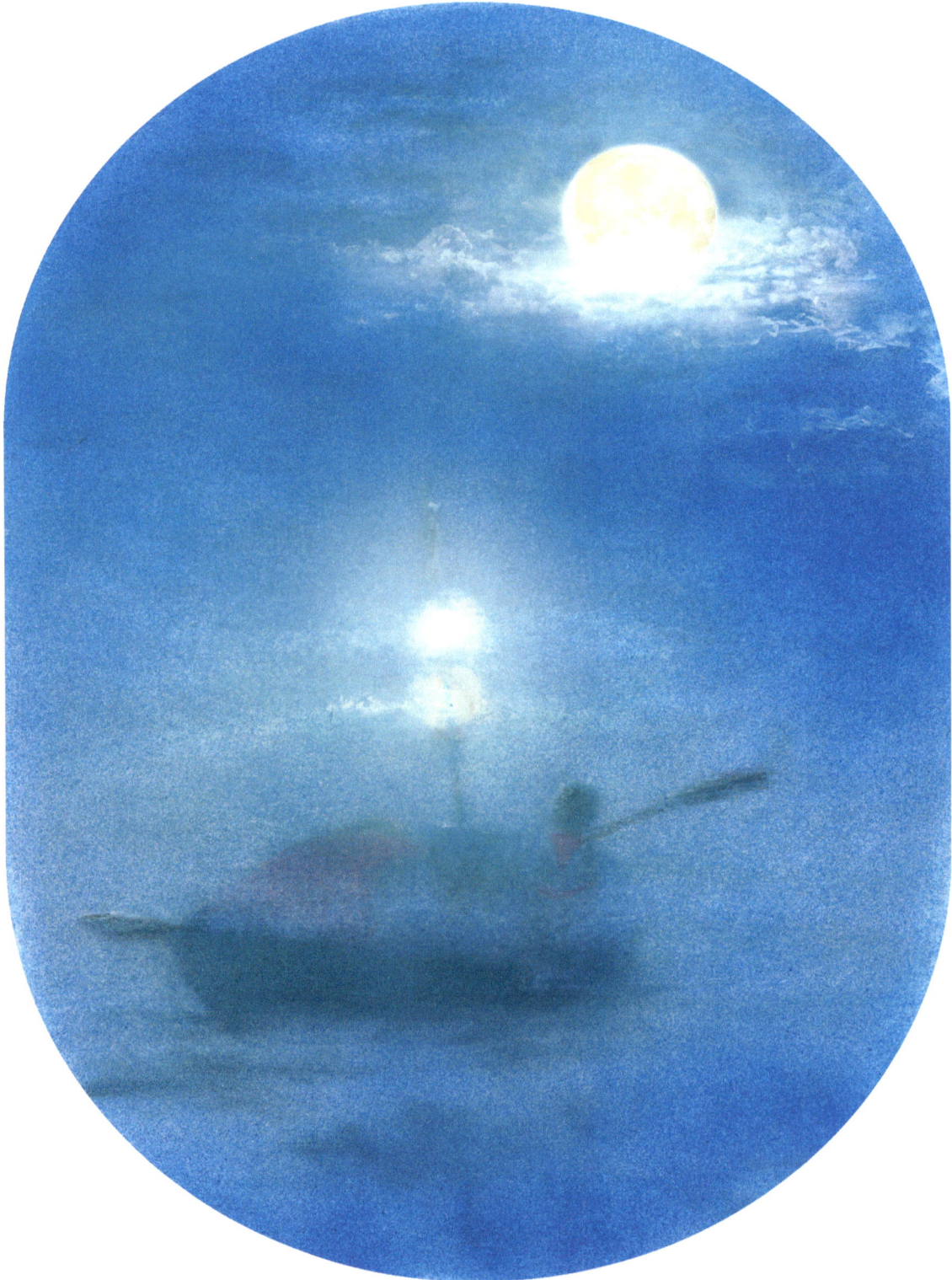

Evening came quickly preceded by fog. Their
cell phones went dead so, no calls, texts, or blogs!

Bedtime arose. They were scared, tired, and cold.
The sun came up fast, and the new day was bold.
Sofat was sorry for what he had done.
Sobrat forgave him. The morning was fun.

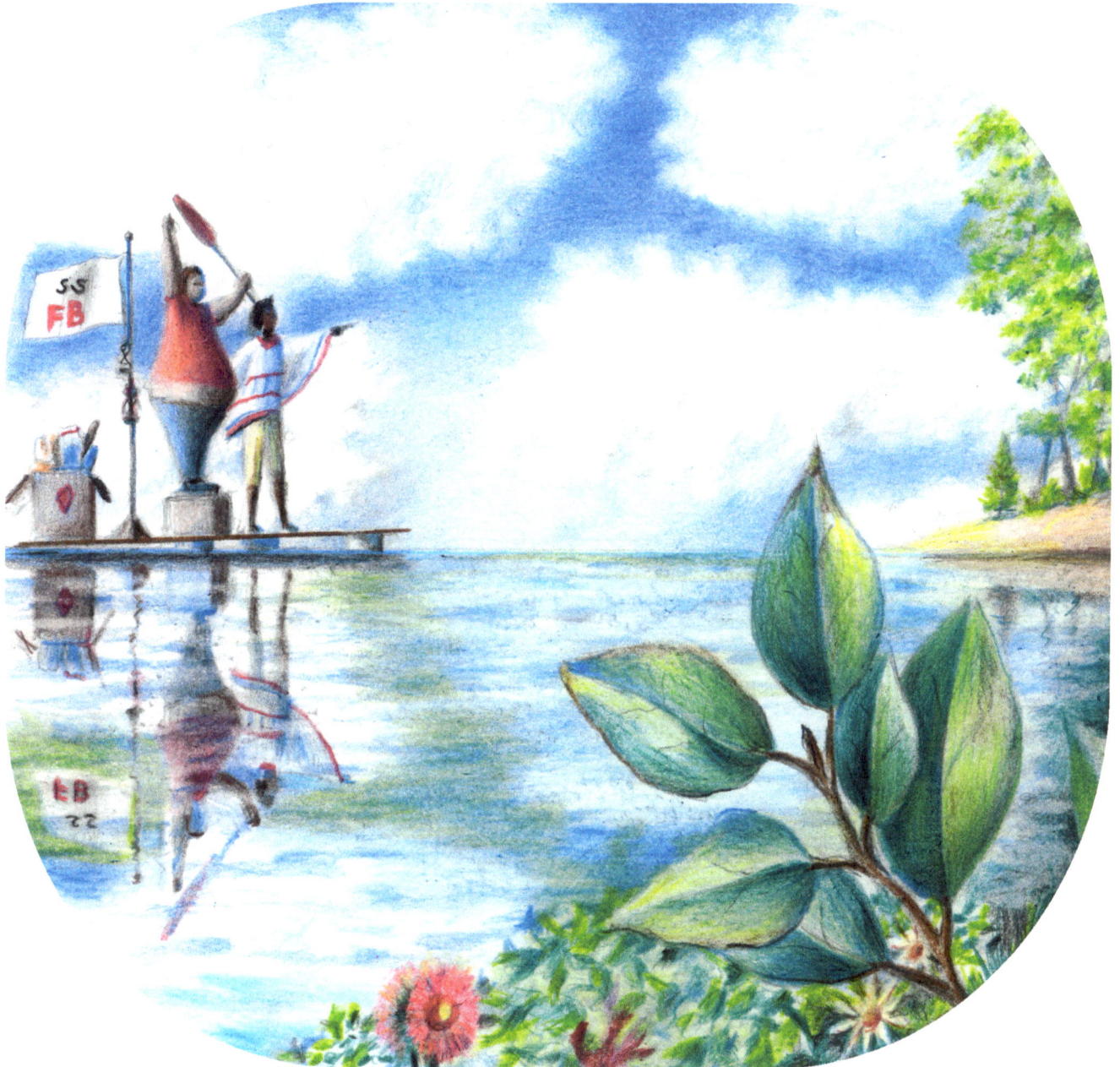

An island was spotted. The raft they did land.
This place had large trees, lush plants, and white sand.
As they walked through the woods, their mouths opened
wide. This was better than new apps or sitting inside!

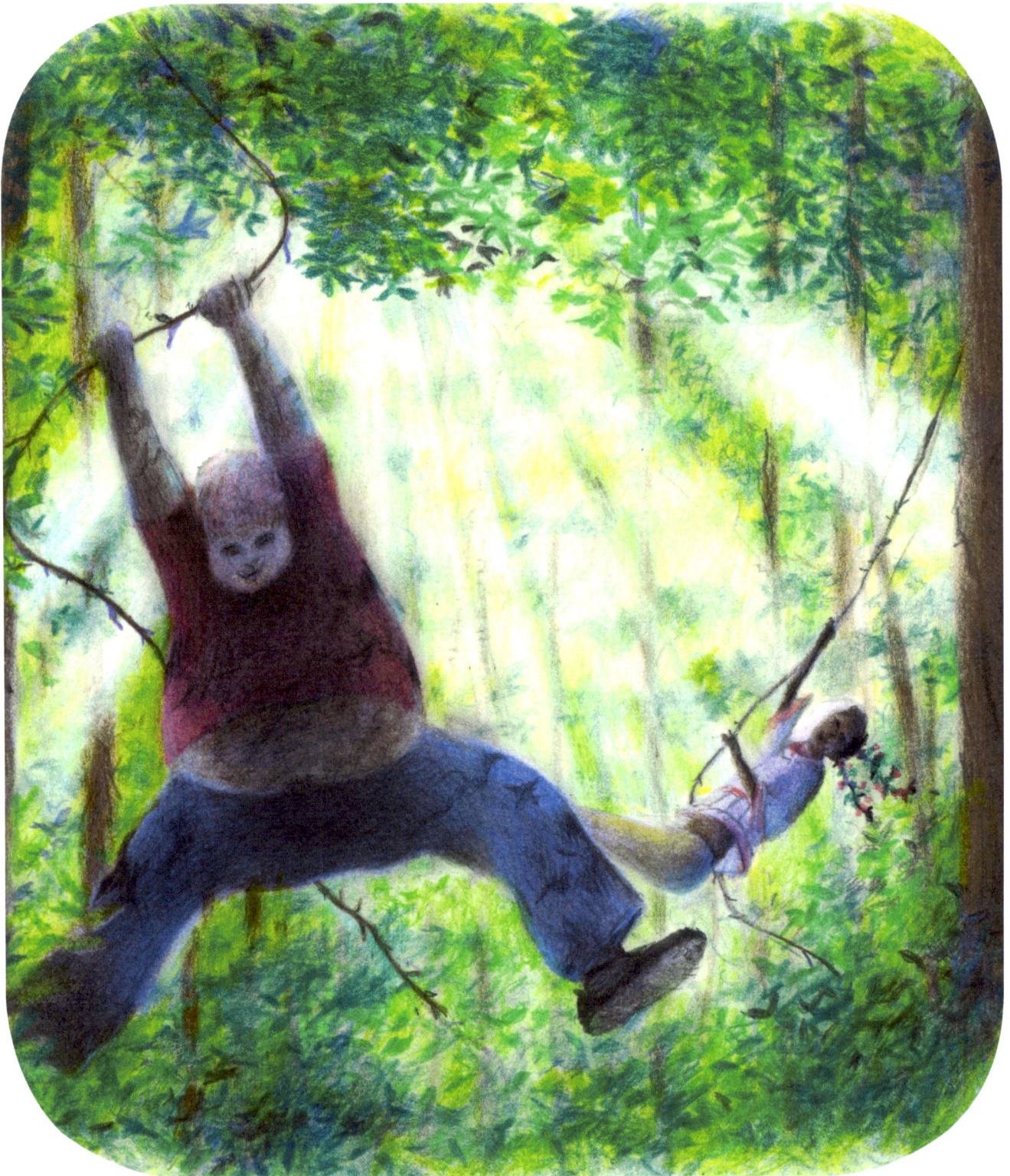

Some trees had plump apples and others great fruit.
They tasted fresh squeezed. Their taste buds did suit.
While climbing up branches and swinging on vines
they didn't miss videos, billboards, or signs.

The rocks, trees, and flowers there, had
awesome features; but this isle was home
for hundreds of creatures.

Raccoons, birds, and squirrels were high in
the limbs. Small chipmunks scurried
and big ducks took swims.

After moving some logs and rolling some stones,
insects were spied there in colorful tones.

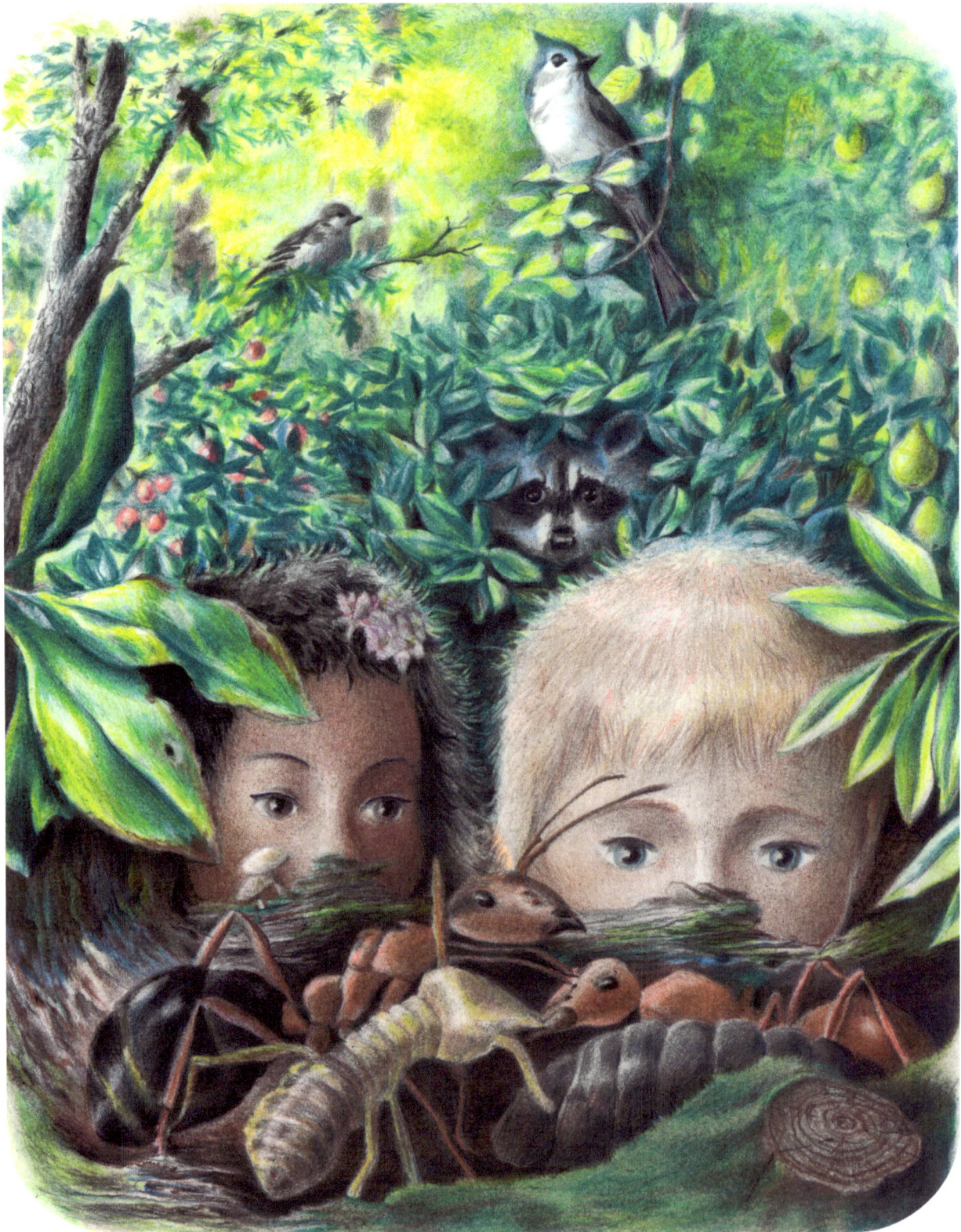

Family and friends were missed when they parted
but wow, what they'd learned; things were
just getting started!

Much fun had been had, so they lost track of time.
The days turned to weeks, then to months, how sublime.

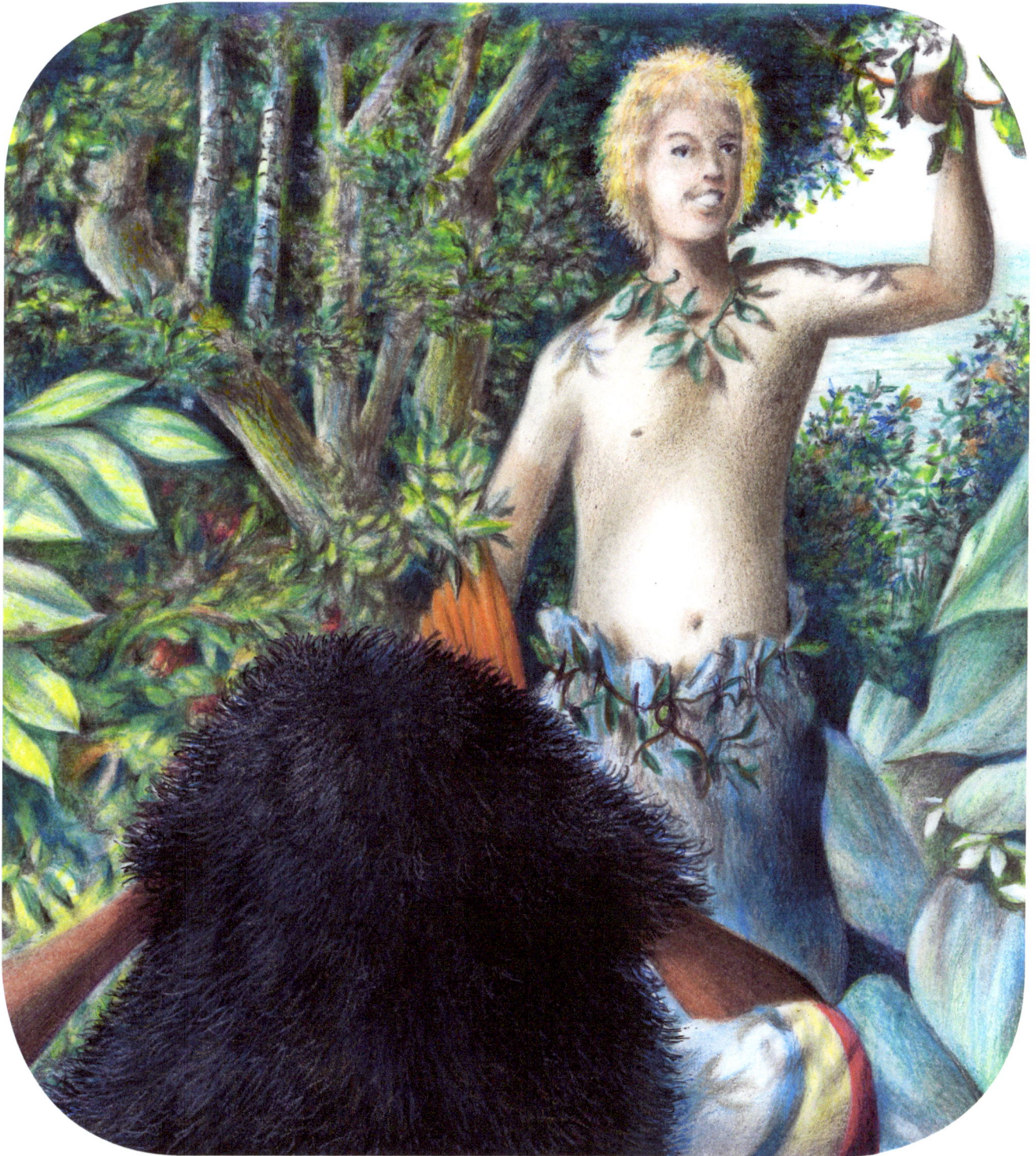

"We were born to do this," now thin Sofat said.
"I am stronger and leaner from toenails to head."

As our friends played one morning a chopper flew by.
At first it was high, then low in the sky. It hovered
down slowly, then sat on the sand. Their parents jumped
out and toward them they ran.

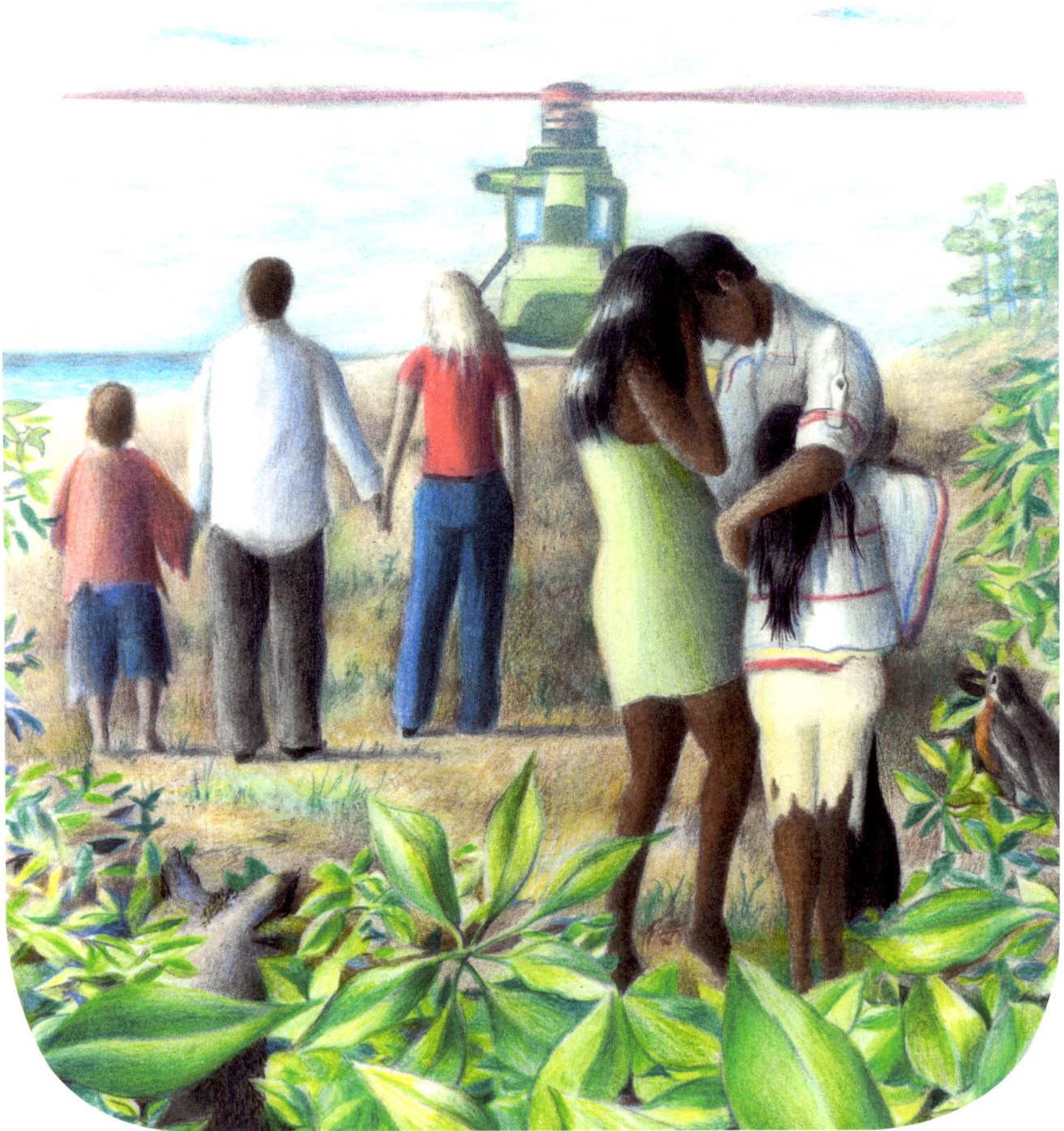

The reunion was great as they all hugged and cried.
They jumped in the copter all ready to ride.

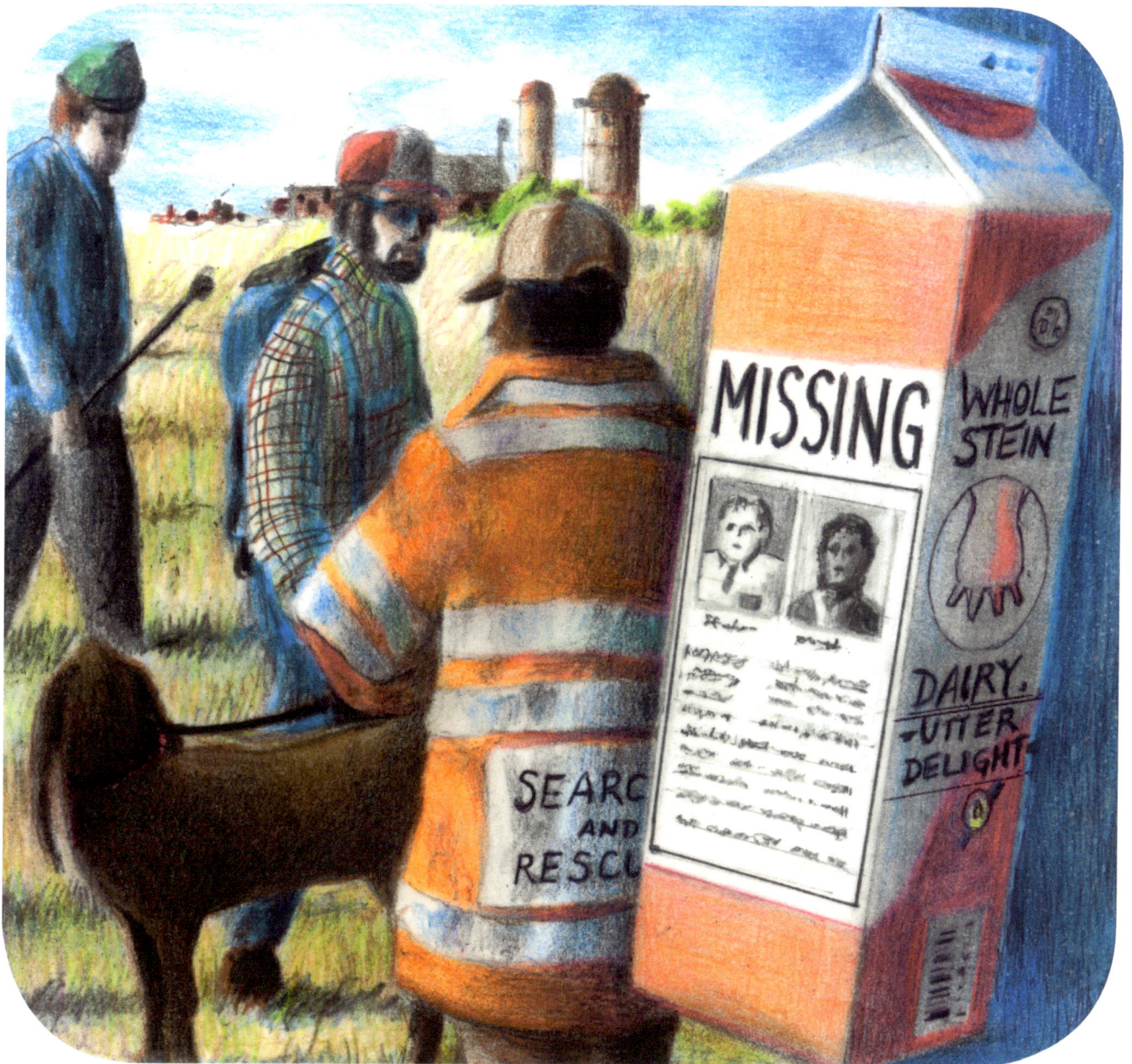

Their folks then told them how worried they'd been.
"We searched for you two, for weeks without end.

On cartons of milk, your pictures were posted and
many search parties were funded and hosted."

The parents, so proud of their kids who had grown,
could hardly believe they were ones they had known.

Now, Sobrat and Sofat a much wiser pair, decided
to take what they'd learned and to share. They went
back to school so much sharper and nice; both
yearning to give fellow students advice.

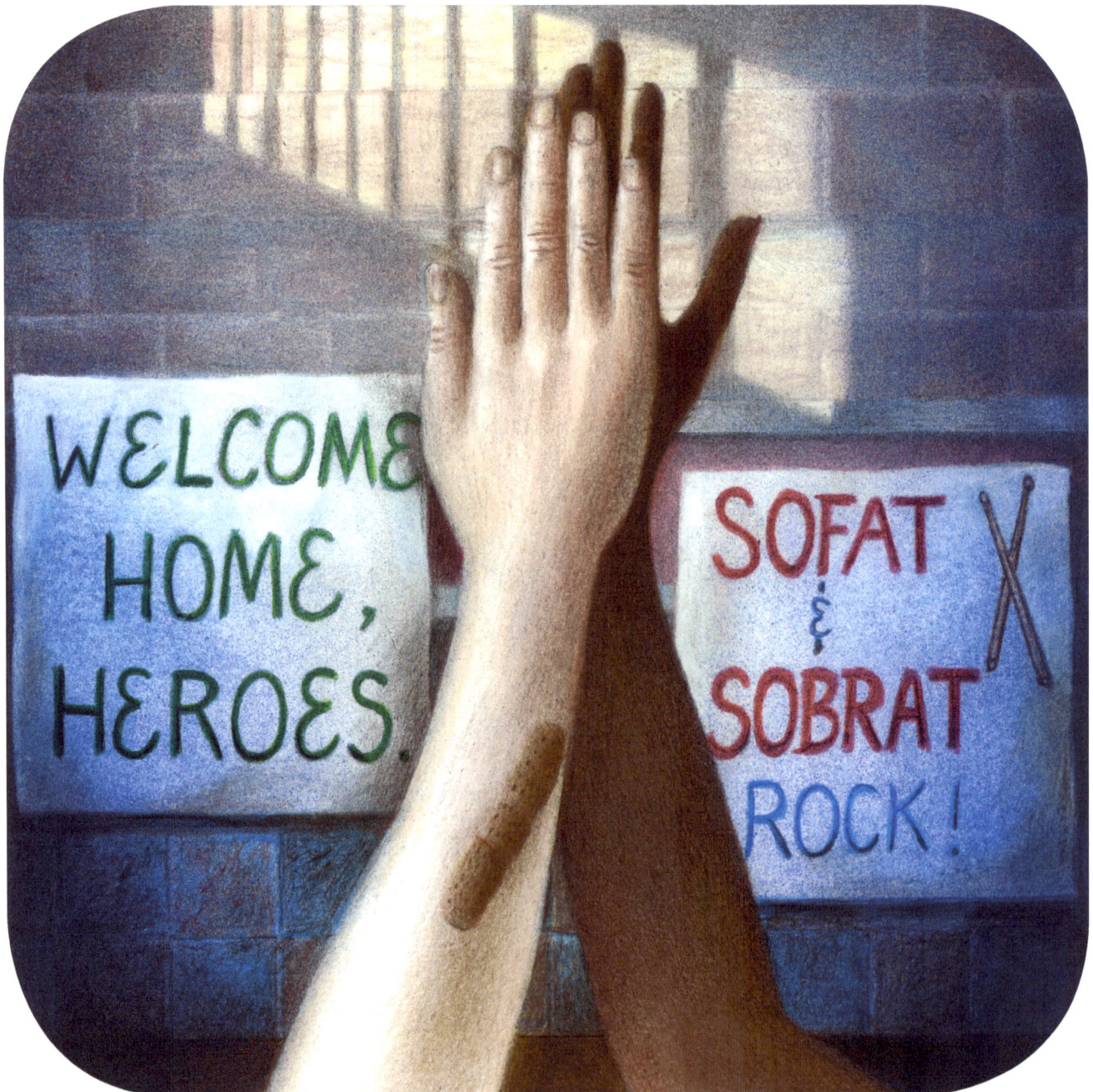

While standing up high and ready to speak,
the place was so quiet, you heard their shoes squeak

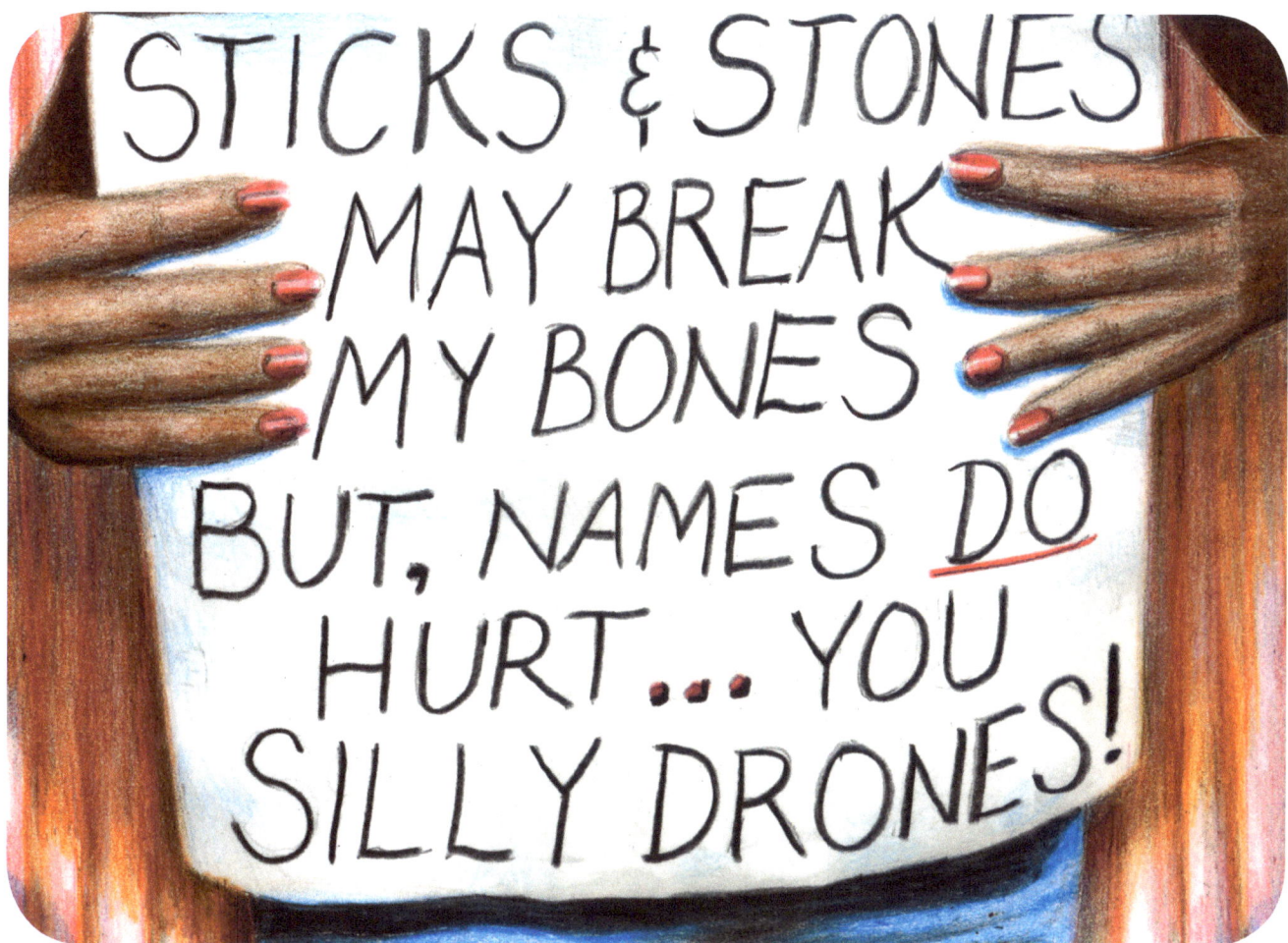

STICKS & STONES MAY BREAK MY BONES BUT, NAMES DO HURT... YOU SILLY DRONES!

Sobrat spoke loudly. Her intention was clear.
She wanted the gang in the huge room to hear.

"Don't bully your friends or even your foes, or
you will receive a big punch in the nose! I was
just joking," she said with a laugh. "We seriously
wanted to show you a path."

"The path that I speak of will bring you more joy,
than harboring hatred or craving that toy. Electronic
tools are part of life now, but we must find a balance
and keep it somehow."

Sofat then spoke with conviction and poise. The crowd got excited and made lots of noise. "Seems most of us now just sit, chew, and talk. We were meant to eat well, stretch, run, jump, and walk."

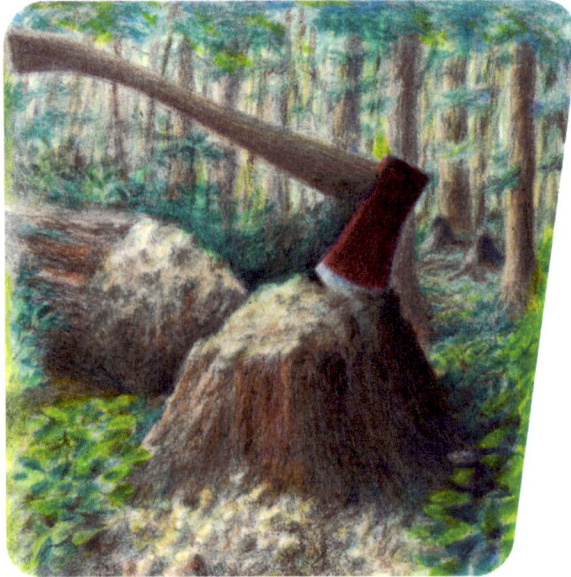

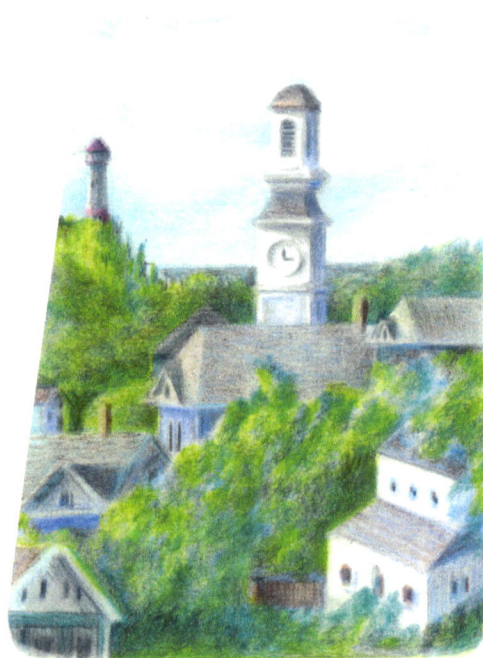

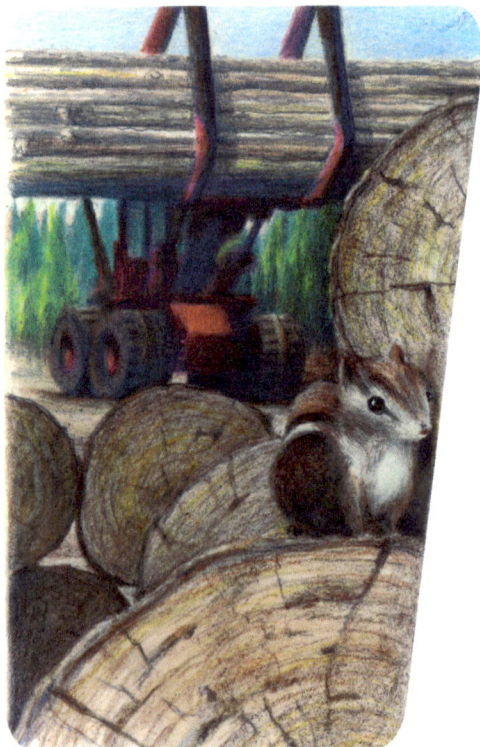

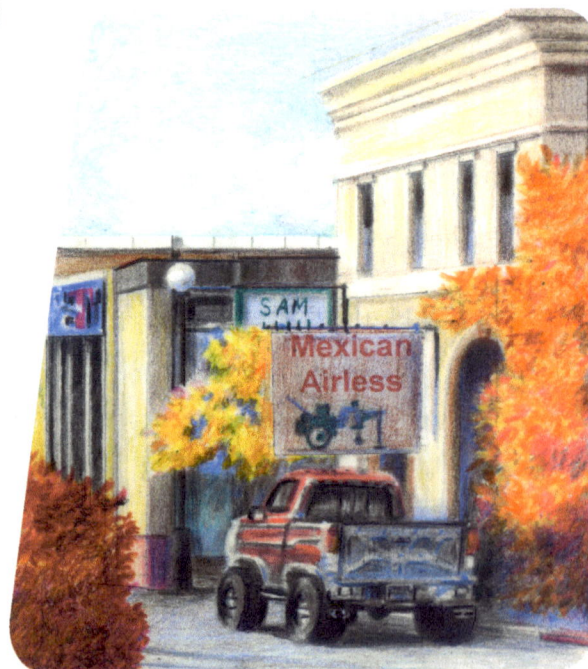

"The earth has been cleared where trees used to stand. Now homes, shops and streets exist there as planned."

"Spend more time outdoors, and visit the woods.
Hang in a forest instead of your hoods."

"If you waste a bright day all snug in the sack, you'll
surely regret it. That day won't be back! Life is
too short to be idle and lazy. Act on good dreams,
have fun, and go crazy!"

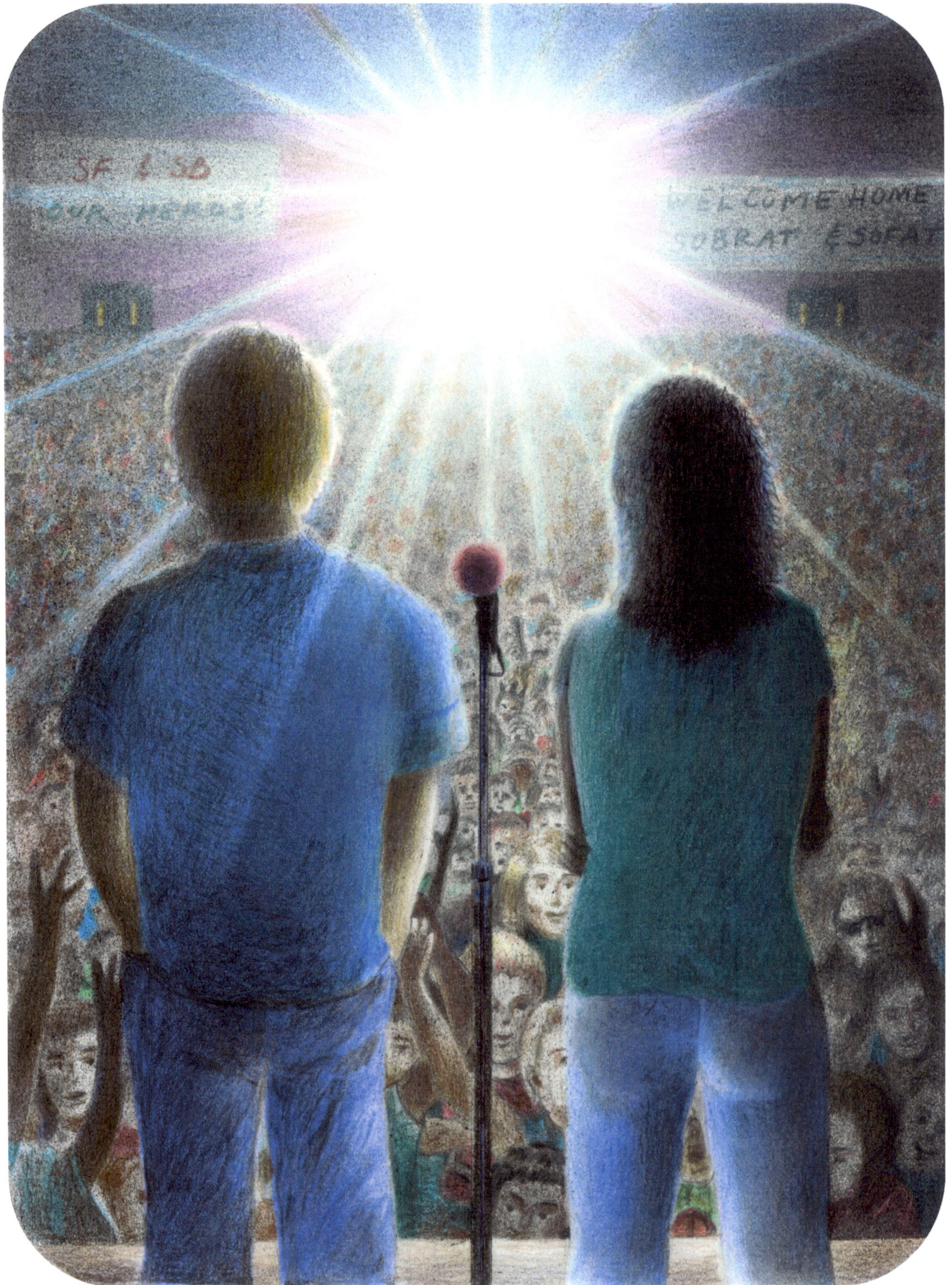

Sobrat stood up with more things to say.
"Please stick around and don't go away.
With most kids today, it's all about ME.
Let's flip that around and make it a WE."

"Just as important, remember this rule. It's
something they can't really teach you in school.
Things have a place, but they're not human beings.
To be truly happy, treat others like kings."

Their speech finally ended, so friends went away;
more enlightened, inspired, and ready to play. As
the story now closes, please heed their advice.

Sofat was **So-fit** and . . .

Sobrat, So-nice!

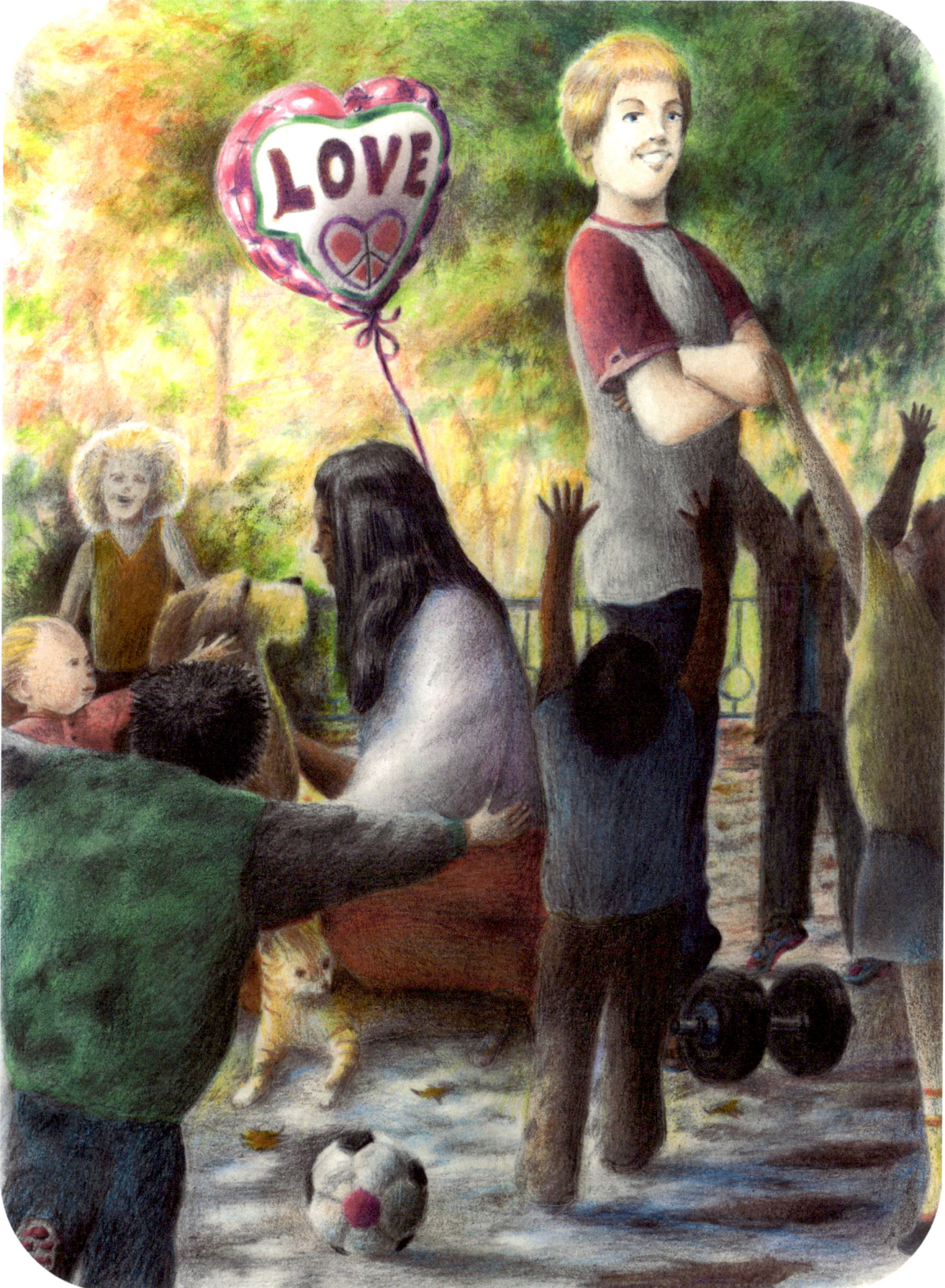

Acknowledgements

My sincere appreciation to the following individuals whose knowledge and efforts contributed to the creation of this book.

Charles and Nancy Clark......................................Editors

Suzanne LaValley-Hines.............................Layout Artist

Stephen Fitzgerald............................. PDF File Creator

Kathryn Evans..Tech Support

Hand Models
(Front Cover)

Michelle Bedes...Sobrat

Ricardo Munoz..Sofat

This book and other titles may be ordered from any neighboorhood bookstore or BarnesandNoble.com